HOW TO #TAOFU FOR EVERYONE

By Rev. Angela Smith

TABLE OF CONTENTS

INTRODUCTION

I define #TaoFu (with or without hashtag (TaoFu)) as the way to respond to vice with the correct corresponding virtue whether the vice is represented as a human vs. self conflict, protagonist individual vs. antagonist individual conflict, human vs. nonhuman animal conflict, or human vs. nature conflict. In my practice, my original arsenal is the shield of love and the sword of truth from which all virtues spring into existence.

The following chapters define the seven deadly sins as vices, provide examples of those vices in action or at play as well as ways to respond to each conscientiously (with virtuous consideration and action). The seven vices explored are commonly called vanity, greed, lust or illicit sexual desire (illicit is defined by Oxford Languages via google.com (Google) as forbidden by law, rules, or custom), envy, gluttony (often referring to luxury, addiction, excess), wrath (often defined as extreme anger, hate, or vengeance), and sloth (laziness).

The Tao of TaoFu is taken from the meaning of Tao (though none really exists, Shikata Ga Nai (Japanese)) I use, which is defined as "A religion native to China. Its adherents attempt to live according to the Tao — the "Way," which they believe governs the universe." Source: https://www.dictionary.com/browse/taoism And, the Fu of TaoFu is taken from the meaning of Fu (as in Kung Fu, with Fu meaning time spent practicing and studying) I use which is defined as "Kung fu/Kungfu or Gung fu/Gongfu is a Chinese term referring to any study, learning, or practice that requires patience, energy, and time to complete, often used in the West to refer to Chinese martial arts, also known as Wushu. It is only in the late twentieth century, that this term was used in relation to Chinese Martial Arts by the Chinese community." Source: https://www.definitions.net/definition/Kung+Fu One of the ways I understand TaoFu is through the lens of Aikido. For my own practice, I also at times refer to TaoFu as Abstract Aikido. Aikido is defined by Oxford Languages via Google as "a Japanese form of self-defense and martial art that uses locks, holds, throws, and the opponent's own movements." It is a self-defense course I've taken as well.

Some of the examples in the following chapters will be in the form of dialogue. There are three ways for #TaoFu to manifest. TaoFu Positive is the best way and exemplifies honest reason, truth, and virtue. #TaoFu Negative is the worst way and exemplifies dishonesty (including intellectual dishonesty), deception, and vice. Totally #TaoFu is when one responds in kind to #TaoFu Negative and often involves discretion that may include lies of omission.

Recognizing equality and mutual respect for all as equals in the eyes of the governing laws in any jurisdiction is the best way to avoid hypocrisy or check yourself on that particular vice. Hypocrisy can attach or be present in many vicious actions whether legal or not. The easiest way to avoid hypocrisy in any course of speech or action is to consider the impacts such will have on others and if in their shoes how you would respond (thinking, feeling, etc) if on the receiving end of the considered course of speech or action. If you would respond poorly or in a #TaoFu Negative way, then that's the response you should expect even if fortunate enough to have a TaoFu Positive audience.

VANITY

Vanity is first and foremost a symptom of hypocrisy in which the vain exult themselves with delusions of grandeur or superiority. But, in dehumanizing others or deifying oneself, the commitment to inequality and hypocrisy manifests in express and implied attempts to subjugate others to the will of the vanity-afflicted. It is one of the seven deadly sins and a vice traditionally responded to with humbleness and/or humility. Personally I prefer the humorous response, which may involve self-deprecating humor to show my own humbleness along with a loving mock in hopes to humble the vain. Recognizing equality of all people in the eyes of God, the universe, the law, and yourself while remaining mindful of that is how to internally stay humble enough and avoid the dangers associated with vanity.

DIALOGUE: VANITY EXAMPLE

Vanity: Pay me tribute or suffer great harm, possibly even death.

#TaoFu Positive Party: May you be as merciful as I am towards you.

Totally #TaoFu Party: That sounds like extortion. What benefit or reward awaits my tribute? If it is solely temporary relief from the immediate threat, I don't find that particularly rewarding. Extortion is a crime.

#TaoFu Negative Party: Is this a get rich quick scheme and can I get in on it? I could be your enforcer and cause harm or death to any who refuse to pay. What's my cut on that tribute?

Vanity: Mercy is not something I can accept in lieu of a tribute. You can remain in my presence and good graces as your reward if you pay tribute.

#TaoFu Positive Party: Mercy is a virtue. All people of good faith accept virtuous tribute. Virtuous tribute is all I have to give. I shall leave your presence in search of your good graces. I'll return upon discovery.

Totally #TaoFu Party: I'm going to leave too.

#TaoFu Negative Party: Neither of you can leave until you pay tribute. Right? I'll kill you if you take a single step before paying. We'll work out the split later.

Vanity: Fine, I accept the virtuous tribute. But, you can't leave until you pay. I accept your assistance as your tribute, there will be no split.

#TaoFu Positive Party: Liars self-negate. If you accept my mercy, I am free to leave.

Totally #TaoFu Party: You want me to press kidnapping charges on top of extortion? The fact Vanity won't pay for your enforcement pisses you off too? I'd have left already without your reinforcements. Vanity is nothing without you.

#TaoFu Negative Party: I'm getting paid for this, right? I'm being of service and so get a cut of the take. That's the deal, right?

Vanity: You are all free to leave. I'm feeling merciful.

#TaoFu Positive Party: You are welcome and I am pleased to discover your good graces.

Totally #TaoFu Party: Don't be surprised if we never meet again.

#TaoFu Negative Party: Should I follow them and collect? Even if I do, doubt you'll see any of it. You waived your share.

END DIALOGUE

MEDITATIVE QUESTIONS:

With which character in the dialogue would you most like to socialize?

Does the character with which you would most like to socialize represent the character that best represents the role you identify with most, least, or not at all?

Which of the characters would you elect to grant any governing authority?

HUMAN VS. SELF - TAOFU EXERCISE

Practice humbleness whenever you feel inclined to subjugate others (over whom you have no authority at law). If possible, recall a time of great embarrassment for you that you now laugh about or hope to someday. If you ever urinated in your own clothes, even in early childhood/grade school, that should ground you in your own humanity, frailty, fallibility, and potential for good humor and error. The moment you wish to subjugate anyone else, that's vanity tempting you to inequality, hypocrisy, and potentially idolatry. Address your own temptations to vice first so you can be an example for those who haven't mastered self-discipline.

INDIVIDUAL PROTAGONIST VS. INDIVIDUAL ANTAGONIST – TAOFU EXERCISE

Are you the protagonist or the antagonist? If you are vain, you are the antagonist and should refer to the Human vs. Self exercise above. If you are the protagonist engaged in conflict with a vain person not yourself, what is the root cause of the conflict? Are you dependent on the vain person/antagonist? If so, the dependency is what you can address to extract yourself from the conflict by pursuing self-sufficiency (also referred to as independence). Is the vain antagonist dependent on you? If so, are you under any legal obligation (contractual or as a result of legal guardianship) to provide for the vain antagonist? If under no legal obligation, your engagement in the conflict is totally your choice and you are free to walk away or dismiss the antagonist. Vices such as Vanity rarely manifest without at least one of the others in tow. Is a vain desire to dominate based on greed (covetousness), jealousy, or envy? Are you responding in kind by trying to dominate in response or remaining mindful of equality while reinforcing it by remaining firm, respectful, objective, patient, and tolerant? If you can record an entire episode of the conflict and play it back for an audience of peers as well as yourself and the antagonist if willing to participate, do so and see how many people laugh including yourself. Whether laughter ensues or not, the audience feedback should humble all involved who need it.

HUMAN VS. NONHUMAN ANIMAL – TAOFU EXERCISE

Many believe Ancient Egyptians worshipped cats, dogs, and dung beetles (AKA scarabs). This is based on artwork featuring all three not unlike how ancient cave-dwellers depicted buffalo or other wild game on cave walls. One can look at the art of Ancient Egypt and see attempts were made and potentially successful in domesticating and bonding with nonhuman animals. It is very possible Sekhmet was an actual Queen of Egypt who was particularly fond of cats which became her symbol, seal, or signature. I don't believe cats, dogs, nor dung beetles ever assumed idol status (false or not) of their own accord beyond enjoying the benefits of being favored by royals of the day and likely fed better than enslaved humans at the time. Do you humanize Sekhmet as you should and hold Sekhmet as objectively equal in humanity to enslaved humans of the time? Do you believe cats might have magic power or be a living totem to an actual deity? Cats are not vain, they are carnivorous hunters and act instinctively as dominant because they have no natural predators besides the occasional trophy-hunting human and are top of the food chain right after humans at this time. Source: https://www.litter-robot.com/blog/why-felines-are-apex-predators/ It is very possible adapting to living with nonhuman animals and having them as pets and/or security systems resulted in deimatic behavior of Ancient Egyptian royals assuming the posture of those most feared felines. And, that superstition grew out of that and possible dehydration, fever, or hallucinogenic intoxication. In 1820, only 12% of the human population knew how to read and write, let alone fact check. As of 2015, 86% of the human population knows how to read and write. Source: https://ourworldindata.org/literacy So, vanity may lure you into believing cave and tomb drawings hold magical mysteries that you can learn by studying dung beetles that eat and push feces around all day though reportedly are what keeps the world turning, but should know magnetic poles and gravitation are the reason for that. Failing to recognize the sun's gravitational pull of the earth as the reason for the earth's rotation to embrace the belief that the dung beetle is the reason is vanity in the form of delusions of grandeur. If you laughed, you successfully completed this exercise. (And, yes, a smile counts.)

HUMAN VS. NATURE – TAOFU EXERCISE

The situation to be contemplated in this exercise is in dialogue format between two human beings. Your task is to determine for yourself whether vanity or ignorance is the primary problem.

DIALOGUE

Inquirer: Do you honestly believe killing one or two humans in some sacrificial rite will prevent a volcanic eruption by appeasing a deity that is the volcano/mountain or controls it?

Tribal Leader: I don't know, last time there was an earthquake there was smoke on the mountain and we threw a couple of virgins in so there was no more earthquake for quite a while. It worked. One time we had no virgins and it erupted taking out our entire village while many of us were away hunting and gathering. We won't make that mistake again. This is why chastity is so important.

Inquirer: Correlation doesn't imply causation. Have you successfully averted any other natural disasters like monsoons or tsunamis or do you appease sky deities through other means? How much influence over deities do you claim to have and what is the evidence of this?

Tribal Leader: Unfortunately, learning that virgins may be sacrificed results in less chastity even when the lives of our entire village are at stake. We assume this angers all deities and this is why we hope animal sacrifices like sacrificing thousands of frogs in Bihar satisfy the rain/sky gods. Earthquakes trigger tsunamis so sacrificing virgins is still the go to on that.

Inquirer: The last flood in Bihar to my knowledge occurred in 2019 and people died in floods in Bihar every year from 1979 through 2019. The frog sacrifice took place in 2018. Source: https://www.business-standard.com/article/news-ians/frog-sacrifice-in-rain-starved-bihar-118071900667_1.html Have you ever studied geography, meteorology, or geology? I honestly think you should so you understand the actual causes of the natural disasters you fear. You may also wish to study natural disaster preparedness to help save as many as possible by planning ahead since often natural disasters are cyclical and even predictable.

Tribal Leader: I don't trust you. Your presence here is angering the gods. Are you a virgin? I shall warn my people to avoid you. You bring great misery and displease our gods.

Inquirer: Will any virgin do or do they need to be from your tribe? I'm not a virgin so wouldn't make a good sacrifice. I'm happily married. My wife asked me to visit your village because she was told you are a wise elder with a special elixir she wanted to try. I looked into it and thought I'd open with my own inquiry. What's in this elixir?

Tribal Leader: It is very special and only for our tribe. I can't give any to you nor your wife. You wouldn't understand the ingredients and it has to be taken as part of a ceremony.

Inquirer: I'm a bit of a botanist familiar enough with chemistry and cooking. My wife suffers terrible food allergies, I'd need to know what's in it and so would she. She'd likely be game for any ceremony at any cost to try that elixir.

Tribal Leader: I can't disclose our secrets to outsiders. Send your wife here alone with $10,000 US in cash and we'll perform the ceremony and she'll consume the elixir. If she tells you our secrets, the elixir won't work. She'll be in breach of her sacred pact as an honorary member of our tribe if she reveals anything.

END DIALOGUE

MEDITATIVE QUESTIONS:

If you were the inquirer would you support or protest your wife's interest and/or further pursuit of the elixir?

Is the tribal leader suffering vanity? Do you think it may be indicative of delusions of grandeur (symptom of vanity) to claim you can stop a natural disaster by sacrificing people or animals to deities you believe or claim control such phenomena?

Do you believe the inquirer is reasonable and open-minded? Do you believe the tribal leader is reasonable and open-minded? What about the inquirer's wife?

If you lived in a society that sacrificed virgins how quickly would you seek to lose your virginity?

FINAL THOUGHT: Ancient Aztecs married as young as 8 years old. Source: https://users.pop.umn.edu/~rmccaa/NAHUAEN3/nacolhst.htm It seems to go beyond ignorance to establish a policy that would result in children having children. The choice of the tribal leader to ignore or avoid learning more rather than experience disillusionment and enlightenment is a willful act. It remains up to you to determine if vanity or ignorance is the greater obstacle. That is the exercise.

GREED

I define the vice of Greed as the opposite of Generosity. Generosity is defined as being synonymous with Magnanimous, which is defined by Oxford Languages via Google as "generous or forgiving, especially toward a rival or less powerful person." Greed is also referred to as Avarice in terms of the seven deadly vices/sins. Avarice is defined by Oxford Languages via Google as "extreme greed for wealth or material gain." And, Greed itself is defined by Oxford Languages via Google as "intense and selfish desire for something, especially wealth, power, or food."

DIALOGUE: GREED EXAMPLE

Generosity: You are welcome to help yourself to anything on those two tables, but the other two are reserved.

Greed: I'm going to take whatever I want without respect nor regard for generosity.

Generosity: I need you to leave, but you can take what you like from the unreserved tables when you go. The other two are display tables that belong to someone else. They will prosecute you for theft.

Greed: I'll risk it. No risk, no reward.

END DIALOGUE

MEDITATIVE QUESTIONS:

With which character in the dialogue would you most like to socialize?

Does the character with which you would most like to socialize represent the character that best represents the role you identify with most, least, or not at all?

Which of the characters would you elect to grant any governing authority?

HUMAN VS. SELF - TAOFU EXERCISE

Whenever you want or demand more than you are legally due, imagine your response to someone wanting or demanding more than you are willing or able to offer (lawfully or not). That is the response you should expect to your own wishes where no one is legally obligated to grant them.

INDIVIDUAL PROTAGONIST VS. INDIVIDUAL ANTAGONIST – TAOFU EXERCISE

Please begin this exercise by (re-)reading "DIALOGUE: GREED EXAMPLE" above on this page. Who is the protagonist? Who is the antagonist? Is the antagonist willfully blind or recklessly disregarding and disrespecting the autonomy and rights of others? As with Vanity, Greed also involves hypocrisy. If in Generosity's position, how would you handle it? #TaoFu Positive, #TaoFu Negative, or Totally #TaoFu? This exercise is intended to help all be more self-aware.

HUMAN VS. NONHUMAN ANIMAL – TAOFU EXERCISE

Beavers cut down 200 trees a year each to build structures for their habitat. Source: https://ed.fnal.gov/entry_exhibits/beaver/beaver.html One lumber/timber company in Mississippi suffered a $215 million loss as a result of beaver interference in one year. Source: https://digitalcommons.usu.edu/cgi/viewcontent.cgi?article=1187&context=hwi Would you consider the beavers greedy? If you were the lumber company that suffered the loss, what would you do? Would you exterminate the beavers? As a consumer, would you pay more for wood and paper products if it meant the beavers get to live?

HUMAN VS. NATURE – TAOFU EXERCISE

For this exercise, imagine you are a gardener or one of the plants involved. The black walnut tree uses chemical warfare to suppress and kill the pine tree, tomato, eggplant, and potato. Source: https://www.gardeningknowhow.com/garden-how-to/info/allelopathic-plants.htm The pine tree responds with a chemical attack of its own. Whichever one wins will ultimately consume the remains of the loser. They both attack what some refer to as weeds, as does the gardener. Is the winner greedy?

FINAL THOUGHT: What does equality mean to you? Thank you for buying this book or to the person who gave it to you as a gift. Whether a gift or not, thank you for your time in reading it. I couldn't afford a $215 million loss ever, let alone in one year. Damage caused by beavers are considered acts of God/nature to most insurance companies. It seems doubtful, though possible, that entire loss could be recovered or neutralized at tax time. Self-defense is natural.

LUST

Lust is unlawful sexual desire, which varies somewhat by region, culture, and jurisdiction. It is a crime to use a vibrator/dildo in Alabama, whether alone or with a partner. Source: https://www.law.ua.edu/acrcl/files/2017/04/ITS_A_DILDO.pdf Alabama is the only state that makes masturbation a crime in itself.

DIALOGUE: LUST EXAMPLE

Inquirer: Have you ever committed rape by fraud/deceit?

Lustful Party #1: I tell people I'm on birth control to get them in bed. I'm not on birth control. Is that rape?

Lustful Party #2: I was charged with rape in Sweden for "stealthing" or failing to wear a condom when I said I would.

Inquirer: Have you ever committed rape by force/coercion?

Lustful Party #1 and #2: No. Never.

Lustful Party #3: I once told my boyfriend if he didn't go down on me, I'd kick him out and break up with him.

Lustful Party #4: Yes, but mercifully killed the "victim".

END DIALOGUE

MEDITATIVE QUESTIONS:

With which character in the dialogue would you most like to socialize?

Does the character with which you would most like to socialize represent the character that best represents the role you identify with most, least, or not at all?

Which of the characters would you elect to grant any governing authority?

HUMAN VS. SELF - TAOFU EXERCISE

If you masturbate in a jurisdiction where that is legal, check local laws before traveling. Osama bin Laden encouraged jihadists to masturbate. Source: https://nypost.com/2017/02/07/osama-bin-laden-was-fine-with-jihadists-masturbating/ It is difficult to imagine anyone more conservative than a jihadist, but Alabama seems to have it covered.

INDIVIDUAL PROTAGONIST VS. INDIVIDUAL ANTAGONIST – TAOFU

EXERCISE

The antagonist is a rapist. Are you a rapist? Rape by fraud is a federal crime in the USA. Source: 10 U.S. Code § 920 - Art. 120.

HUMAN VS. NONHUMAN ANIMAL – TAOFU EXERCISE

Bestiality is legal in Wyoming, West Virginia, New Mexico, and Hawaii. Source: https://newrepublic.com/article/160448/meat-bestiality-artificial-insemination There is no federal law in the US criminalizing bestiality. Source: http://jaapl.org/content/early/2019/05/16/JAAPL.003836-19 Seals (AKA Sea Lions) rape penguins. Source: https://www.cbsnews.com/news/strange-but-true-seals-found-sexually-assaulting-penguins/ Is such behavior symptomatic of mental illness in your opinion? Would you rather be convicted of a crime and serve a definite sentence or found insane with an indefinite commitment in a psychiatric hospital for the criminally insane?

HUMAN VS. NATURE – TAOFU EXERCISE

Do you suffer seasonal allergies? Has your vehicle ever been covered in pollen in the morning? Pollens are tiny plant penises. Source: https://www.studyfinds.org/pollen-tube-science-finally-unlocked-secrets-behind-natures-largest-erection/ There is no law against it. Do you consider allergies or your car covered in pollen sexual assault or rape? Is it more the lack of intent to harm or that everyone living outside of a bubble has experienced it that helps you forgive?

FINAL THOUGHT: I am a sexual assault survivor. I also suffer seasonal allergies. I find the above exercises helpful and hope you do too.

ENVY

I define the vice of envy as awareness of a deficiency one wishes to hide or increase at the expense of others. Oxford Languages via Google defines "Envy" as "(noun) a feeling of discontented or resentful longing aroused by someone else's possessions, qualities, or luck" and "(verb) desire to have a quality, possession, or other desirable attribute belonging to (someone else)." Personal integrity and respect for self and others is how I respond to envy. I recognize dishonesty as a form of disrespect.

DIALOGUE: ENVY EXAMPLE

Server: Sorry, we just sold out. Would you like to try something else from the menu?

Envy: Make more. I'll wait.

Server: There is no more. Vanity and Greed took the last of it.

Envy: I can wait.

Server: It was a one-time only special today and there are no plans to make more at this time. It attracted too many vicious people. Something else perhaps?

Envy: Anywhere else I can get it? Where were Vanity and Greed headed?

Server: Sloth's house. But, Greed doesn't share.

Envy: I just checked Google and you were the only place to get that. I hate Vanity and Greed. They ruin everything.

END DIALOGUE

MEDITATIVE QUESTIONS:

Is Envy's main problem impatience, arriving too late/lack of due diligence, or Greed and Vanity?

Are Envy and Sloth the offspring of Vanity and Greed? If so, do you favor any over the others? Is Vanity responsible for the previous question?

HUMAN VS. SELF - TAOFU EXERCISE

If you feel tempted to envy, meditate on the fact that your annual equal share of Global Gross Domestic Product is valued at $10,925.73 (c.e. 2020s, see https://www.cope.church/10grand.png). If you receive equal to that in goods, services, and financial compensation, you are #TaoFu Positive when it comes to hypocrisy in the event you support any economic system other than free market capitalism. If you receive more than that in goods, services, and financial compensation, yet favor socialism or communism, if you do not redistribute all goods, services, and financial compensation you hold over $10,925.73 annually, you are a hypocrite and need to address that by embracing capitalism or redistributing your wealth to align with actual available resources in consideration of the entire human population. Hypocrisy is #TaoFu Negative.

INDIVIDUAL PROTAGONIST VS. INDIVIDUAL ANTAGONIST – TAOFU EXERCISE

Envy often manifests with Sloth as conjoined twins, but not always. For this exercise, envy is the vice of the antagonist. Does the envious party usually get exactly what they want with little to no effort beyond communicating it? If so, the envious party is accustomed to that level of service and may be unaware of how sloth plays any role when they don't get what they want when they want it. College graduates in the US earn an average of $20.85 per hour and/or $43,367/year. Source: https://www.ziprecruiter.com/Salaries/College-Grads-Salary High school graduates in the US earn an average of $19.34/hour and/or $40,223/year. Source: https://www.ziprecruiter.com/Salaries/High-School-Graduate-Salary--in-Washington So, with one's own earned income in a free market, one can acquire what they want if it is in their current budget or save up for it if what they want is a product or service available in the free market. Determining whether what appears to be envy or sloth is vicious or a symptom of developmental/learning disability can be difficult. And, neither of those labels are what Vanity consider particularly flattering. If regression manifests such as throwing a tantrum, pouting, crying, or whining at an otherwise mature age for most, this suggests developmental disability. If not, then you might be dealing with someone some professionals would call a malignant narcissist (criminal mind). Considering the facts and reasons for envy's dissatisfaction should resolve it for the person of average intelligence or greater and reveal whether or not some developmental disability went undiagnosed and unaddressed by neglectful or vain primary caregivers prior to the envious reaching age of majority. If the envious party wants to travel in space, they will need to pay at least $50,000 for one seat on a commercial space flight. Source: https://worldview.space/flight-reserve/ If they cannot afford that, they will need to become part of a crew whether through NASA or private commercial space travel providers. Two years of training at minimum to become an astronaut with NASA. Source: https://www.nasa.gov/feature/frequently-asked-questions-0/#:~:text=The%20astronaut%20candidates%20will%20undergo,upon%20selection%20for%20a%20flight . Is the need for instant gratification envy's actual problem? Patience is the solution for envy and diligence is the solution for sloth.

HUMAN VS. NONHUMAN ANIMAL – TAOFU EXERCISE

As stated in the section on Vanity, cats will replace humans as top of the food chain on earth in the event humans are wiped out and cats survive. All other species on earth capable of envy, envy humanity's position at the top of the food chain. Do you idolize cats? Do you believe cats envy you? Some humans support the extinction of all carnivorous animals including cats. Source: https://www.theatlantic.com/culture/archive/2010/09/should-we-kill-off-the-carnivores/340037/ Meditate on that.

HUMAN VS. NATURE – TAOFU EXERCISE

Plants such as trees and flowers require nutrient rich soil/fertilizer which when organic can contain decayed/dead plants, nonhuman animal corpses, and human corpses. Sources: https://earthfuneral.com/ and https://www.pennington.com/all-products/fertilizer/resources/what-is-organic-fertilizer Though plants are relatively stationary, their diet is one of a scavenger. Plants require the death of other living things in order to live. Do you envy the stationary life of plants? Do you believe plants envy humans? Plants are not picky eaters and potentially unaware that any living thing gets a choice. Meditate on that.

FINAL THOUGHT: If you are unhappy with what you have, imagine not having it.

GLUTTONY

Oxford Languages via Google defines "Gluttony" as "habitual greed or excess in eating." Other definitions from various sources have included luxury, excessive alcohol consumption, and addiction when defining Gluttony. Moderation is how I protect myself from the vice of gluttony.

DIALOGUE: GLUTTONY EXAMPLE

Glutton #1: I need more money so I can gamble so I can have more money.

Glutton #2: I need a ride to the liquor store because I lost my license.

Glutton #3: I need a butler or personal chef to prepare and bring me food because I can no longer walk as a result of self-induced disability.

END DIALOGUE

MEDITATIVE QUESTIONS:

With which character in the dialogue would you most like to socialize?

Does the character with which you would most like to socialize represent the character that best represents the role you identify with most, least, or not at all?

Which of the characters would you elect to grant any governing authority?

HUMAN VS. SELF - TAOFU EXERCISE

Have you ever indulged in or been tempted to excess or extremes? If you indulged, did you find the risks/harm to outweigh any benefit you gained from it? Would you have everyone practice gluttony/excess? If you have indulged in excess but would not advise it for everyone, is that leading by example? Meditate on that.

INDIVIDUAL PROTAGONIST VS. INDIVIDUAL ANTAGONIST – TAOFU EXERCISE

The situation to be contemplated in this exercise is in dialogue format between two human beings. Your task is to determine for yourself what vices already covered in addition to gluttony are present.

DIALOGUE

Party #1: I'm not losing the house over this shit. You need to stop.

Party #2: It's my house too and a free country.

Party: #1: When is the last time you paid the mortgage? Never?

Party #2: That has nothing to do with it. I take care of all of it.

Party #1: Without me, there would be nothing for you to take care of in the first place. How much do you owe?

Party #2: Just write a check out to me or "cash" for $5000 and I'll work out the rest.

END DIALOGUE

MEDITATIVE QUESTIONS:

With which character in the dialogue would you most like to socialize?

Does the character with which you would most like to socialize represent the character that best represents the role you identify with most, least, or not at all?

Which of the characters would you elect to grant any governing authority?

HUMAN VS. NONHUMAN ANIMAL – TAOFU EXERCISE

The runt of a litter of puppies was excluded or blocked by siblings from accessing sufficient mother's milk to avoid malnutrition causing health issues. If you adopted this puppy, he/she may actually need to eat more and exhibit food insecurity throughout his/her life. Behavioral issues may involve hoarding. Is the puppy a glutton?

HUMAN VS. NATURE – TAOFU EXERCISE

Fungi destroyed an entire forest by engaging in excess. Source: https://news.berkeley.edu/2011/08/05/fungi-helped-destroy-forests-during-mass-extinction-250-million-years-ago/ . Are anti-fungal responses punishment enough? Is it right to punish fungi? Can fungi learn from those who lead by example? Meditate on that.

FINAL THOUGHT: Is gluttony only an issue for the envious?

WRATH

I define wrath as unmerciful anger or hate. All the other vices, including wrath, tempt others to wrath. I personally tend to respond to it with a sense of humor.

DIALOGUE: WRATH EXAMPLE

WRATH: If this program locks this file, makes it read only, or claims it was corrupted and lost one more time, I'm going to destroy the machine.

Inquirer: Has it been happening a lot? Have you tried troubleshooting?

END DIALOGUE

MEDITATIVE QUESTIONS:

Is Wrath's biggest issue in the dialogue impatience, ignorance, or sloth?

Would exercising or practicing the virtues of patience and diligence neutralize Wrath?

Is Wrath the vice you empathize with most? If so, do you believe that upsets Vanity?

HUMAN VS. SELF - TAOFU EXERCISE

Think about someone or something you strongly dislike (and/or hate) and challenge yourself to identify/come up with 5 things you like about him/her/it. The purpose of this exercise is to manage your temptation to Wrath (i.e. Hate). If you identify at least one thing you like during this exercise, you've succeeded.

INDIVIDUAL PROTAGONIST VS. INDIVIDUAL ANTAGONIST – TAOFU EXERCISE

When someone approaches you with hate/wrath, if you respond with intention to clear up confusion or make peace then you are #TaoFu Positive. In the same situation, if you respond defensively without escalating tensions, then you are Totally #TaoFu. And, in that same situation, if you escalate then you are #TaoFu Negative. How do you determine who is the protagonist and who is the antagonist? Meditate on that.

HUMAN VS. NONHUMAN ANIMAL – TAOFU EXERCISE

A Shih Tzu named Mollie and a Lhasa Apso named Crystal were companion animals to two separate people living in the same house. This is a true story. Mollie took Crystal's favorite toy which was a stuffed hedgehog dog toy and demolished it in less than 10 minutes. Crystal was devastated. A replacement that was the same toy at market was no consolation. She wouldn't touch it. Mollie had a favorite rubber ball toy that squeaked. She played soccer with it (kind of) all the time. Over a few months Crystal took small bites off that ball whenever she had the chance until it was destroyed. Mollie just played with another ball she liked and didn't seem to care much about the loss of her favorite. As the human companion to either, whose side would you take and would it matter which dog was your companion? Are dogs capable of wrath too?

HUMAN VS. NATURE – TAOFU EXERCISE

Please take a moment to review the greed and gluttony exercises under the same category on pages 11 and 18 respectively. Do allelopathic plants exhibit wrath? What about fungi? Is a tornado to humans the same as a vacuum cleaner to insects? Do you vacuum out of wrath towards any insects that might be killed or disturbed by it? Meditate on that.

FINAL THOUGHT: I find the above helpful in responding to wrath or temptations to wrath and hope you do too.

SLOTH

I don't feel like writing this one. Do it yourself. That is the exercise.

FINAL THOUGHT: Did you need more space? Are you disappointed by this section? Did you see it as a fun opportunity? Did you see it as an opportunity of any kind? Based on your answers to those questions, are you being #TaoFu Positive, Totally #TaoFu, or #TaoFu Negative?

If it isn't true, it isn't love. There are ways to determine if something is true or not. I prefer the scientific method when something is not self-evident. 1 John 4:8 (KJV) "God is love". 1 Corinthians 13:6 (NIV) "Love does not delight in evil but rejoices with the truth." John 8:44 KJV "Ye are of your father the devil...He was a murderer from the beginning, and abode not in the truth, because there is no truth in him. When he speaketh a lie, he speaketh of his own: for he is a liar, and the father of it."

Using the scientific method, begin with a yes or no question where the answer is not self-evident to you and take an affirmative position as your hypothesis and question that position as your test of it. Example:

1. Ask A Yes or No Question: Are over-the-counter dietary/herbal supplements safe to consume?

2. Take A Firm Position/Hypothesis: No, they are not safe to consume.

3. Test The Hypothesis/Research: GNC, Walmart, Walgreens, and Target prosecuted because they sold fraudulent and dangerous supplements that didn't even contain what was on the label. Source: https://well.blogs.nytimes.com/2015/02/03/new-york-attorney-general-targets-supplements-at-major-retailers/

4. Analyze Data and Draw Conclusion: The risk outweighs the alleged benefit.

The quick tip on universalizing your love to the reasonable extent possible is to think of what or who you love most or even more than anything and if someone tempts you to wrath think of your most loved person or object saying or doing the same thing and how you'd respond in such a case, try to respond that way and love is platonic with very few exceptions.

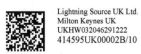

Lightning Source UK Ltd.
Milton Keynes UK
UKHW032046291222
414595UK00002B/10

9 781387 890293